Understanding
Traumatic Brain Injury

*An Essential Guide to Causes,
Symptoms, and Treatment Options
for Individuals with TBI*

By

Isabella White

Table of Contents

Introduction

Traumatic brain injury (TBI) refers to damage to the brain caused by an external physical force. It is one of the most common causes of disability and death worldwide, and anyone can be affected. TBIs occur when a sudden trauma damages brain tissue.

The trauma can result from a jolt or blow to the head that disrupts normal brain function. Alternatively, in more severe cases, the trauma can cause tears, shearing, or bleeding within the brain, which also affects its function.

TBIs can arise from a variety of causes, though the most common are falls, motor vehicle accidents, collisions during sports or recreational activities, and assaults or violence. The resulting injury depends on factors like the amount and type of force, the part of the brain affected, and the individual's age and health. Mild TBIs lead to temporary dysfunction of brain cells. At the same time, more severe injuries produce bruising, torn tissues, bleeding, and other physical damage that can result in long-term complications or death.

When a TBI occurs, the brain goes through both immediate and delayed responses. Initially, the physical trauma causes direct damage by tearing neural connections and blood vessels. Next, secondary injury further harms brain cells through disruptions in blood flow, the release of neurotransmitters, oxidative stress, and inflammation. The consequences of even a mild TBI can persist for weeks, months, or years after the initial injury.

Common effects of TBI include cognitive problems like confusion, memory loss, reduced processing speed, communication impairments, sensory disorders, changes in sleep patterns or mood, and deficiencies in motor control or balance. These issues vary based on factors like injury location and severity. TBI can also increase the long-term risk of neurological disorders such as epilepsy, Parkinson's disease, and Alzheimer's disease.

While anyone is susceptible, certain groups have higher TBI rates and risks. For example, young children, teens, and older adults are more vulnerable to TBIs from falls. Men also experience higher rates of TBI overall. However, proper awareness, preventative measures, and treatment can reduce complications and improve outcomes after a TBI. Ongoing research advances our understanding of how to prevent, assess, and manage TBIs.

The Importance of Understanding TBI

Traumatic brain injury (TBI) is a major health concern that affects millions annually. Gaining a thorough understanding of TBI is crucial for several reasons.

First, awareness empowers both individuals and society. For those living with TBI, knowledge enables them to make informed decisions about treatment and support options. It also allows for setting reasonable expectations for recovery. At a societal level, understanding TBI facilitates the development of better preventative measures, diagnostic tools, therapies, and support systems.

Second, understanding TBI aids in proper recognition and response when an injury occurs. Identifying signs like disorientation, loss of consciousness, vomiting, or amnesia can indicate a TBI right after trauma. Knowing when to seek immediate medical care improves outcomes. Ongoing awareness also helps to notice emerging issues like headaches, sensitivities to light or noise, and cognitive or emotional changes that may appear days or weeks post-injury.

Third, comprehension of TBI facilitates recovery and lowers the risk of repeated injury. Knowledge empowers individuals to advocate for their needs during treatment and rehabilitation. It also allows lifestyle changes to manage residual effects, from adopting brain-healthy nutrition to using devices and strategies that support memory and reduce cognitive fatigue. Additionally, understanding factors that increase vulnerability to TBI helps individuals take protective measures.

Fourth, a clear picture of TBI, its causes, and its impacts promotes the development of better care systems. Insights from individuals living with TBI can inform the delivery of medical, rehabilitative, and community services. Data on trends and risk factors enables prevention initiatives and policy changes. Research expands diagnostics and evidence-based treatment protocols.

Finally, increased understanding reduces stigma. Widespread education diminishes misconceptions of TBI as a singular event with a preset timeline for recovery. Knowledge fosters empathy, demonstrates the spectrum of possible outcomes, and clarifies that effects may linger or evolve. This understanding encourages family, friends, employers, and society to provide ongoing validation and support.

Comprehending key aspects of traumatic brain injury empowers those affected, guides proper response, aids recovery, promotes progress in care systems, and reduces stigma. For clinicians, individuals with TBI, family members, policymakers, and the general public, developing greater knowledge about this complex health issue is vital to improving the lives of millions of people worldwide living with TBI.

The Purpose of this Book

The purpose of this book is to provide an essential, accessible guide to traumatic brain injury (TBI) for those affected and their loved ones. By clearly explaining key aspects of TBI in an easy-to-understand manner, this book aims to empower readers to advocate for their needs, aid recovery, and improve quality of life after a TBI occurs. Specifically, the book serves several key goals:

- **Increase understanding of TBI causes, symptoms, diagnosis, and treatment.** The book presents comprehensive overviews of the common causes of TBI, ranging from accidents to assaults. It outlines acute symptoms and those that may emerge days or weeks later. The book explains standard diagnostic tests and tools used to assess injury severity. It also surveys treatment options and protocols, from emergency care through long-term rehabilitation.

- **Discuss the effects of TBI on daily life.** The book delves into common challenges those with TBI face in cognition, communication, sensory processing, behavior, emotions, and motor skills. It provides strategies and tips for managing these issues at home, work, or school. The content also covers building a support system and asking for accommodations.

- **Explain the recovery process and outcomes.** By exploring potential outcomes across the spectrum and the factors that influence them, this book gives readers realistic insights into the often long and difficult recovery process. Content balances hopefulness with frank discussions of possible long-term complications.

- **Provide research-based guidance for care.** Backed by the latest scientific evidence and clinical standards, the book offers guidance on treatments, lifestyle approaches, and support strategies to aid recovery and minimize residual disability after TBI.

- **Offer resources for finding help and support.** Comprehensive lists of national and local organizations, websites, hotlines, and more enable readers to connect to TBI information, programs, services, and communities.

This empathetic yet informative guide aims to help readers navigate life after TBI with greater clarity, empowerment, and hope by synthesizing medical expertise and personal perspectives. For individuals and families affected by this complex injury, arming oneself with knowledge is key to advocating for needs, accessing quality care, and improving one's path forward. This book aims to provide that valuable understanding and be a trusted resource.

Chapter 1

Causes of Traumatic Brain Injury

Types of Traumatic Brain Injuries

Traumatic brain injuries (TBIs) arise when sudden trauma damages the brain. This damage occurs in two main ways: a closed head injury and a penetrating head injury.

Closed Head Injury:
Closed head injury is the most common type of TBI, accounting for over 80% of cases. As the name suggests, the skull and dura mater remain intact with closed head injuries. These occur when the head accelerates, rapidly decelerates, or collides with an

object. This jolts or shakes the brain inside the skull, stretching and damaging brain cells and blood vessels.

Common causes include falls, motor vehicle accidents, sports collisions, and assaults involving blunt-force trauma. The traumatic acceleration, deceleration, or impact harms the brain through coup and contrecoup effects. Coup injuries occur directly below the area that was struck. Contrecoup injuries happen on the side opposite from the impact. These mechanisms explain why many closed-head TBIs damage frontal and temporal brain regions.

Closed head injuries cover a wide spectrum of severity. Mild cases cause confusion, headaches, and concussion symptoms that resolve within days or weeks. Severe cases can result in bruising, bleeding in the brain, torn nerve fibers, oxygen deprivation, dangerous swelling, and long-term disabilities. Prompt emergency care is vital.

Penetrating Head Injury:
Penetrating head injuries occur when a foreign object pierces through the skull into the brain. Common causes include gunshot wounds, stabbings, and

fragments of shattered skull bone driven inward by high-impact trauma. Penetrating head trauma also happens in vehicle accidents, industrial mishaps, and other situations where high-velocity objects enter the brain.

The path of penetration damages localized brain structures. Temporary cavities, or holes, form around the object. These crush nerve fibers and blood vessels in surrounding areas. Penetrating injuries pose a high risk for hemorrhage, infection, severe swelling, and death. Rapid surgery is required in many cases to remove foreign objects and stop bleeding.

Causes of Traumatic Brain Injury

Traumatic brain injuries (TBIs) can arise from a variety of causes. However, the majority of TBIs result from just a few types of common events. Understanding these frequent causes provides insights into prevention and aids prompt recognition when injury occurs. The four most prevalent causes of TBI are falls, car accidents, sports-related injuries, and violence or assault.

Falls:

Falls are the top cause of TBI overall. They are the leading cause of hospital visits for TBIs across all ages. Falls frequently produce closed-head injuries by slamming the brain against the inside of the skull. Older adults are especially susceptible to falls due to age-related vision loss, weaker bones, the use of medications, and gait/balance issues. Younger children also commonly suffer TBIs from falls, given their developing coordination.

Car Accidents:

Motor vehicle crashes are another frequent cause of head trauma. Car accidents commonly cause closed head injuries—often severe ones—through rapid deceleration, collisions with steering wheels or windows, or ejection from the car. Traumatic brain damage from car crashes includes bruising, bleeding, torn nerve connections, and oxygen deprivation. Using seat belts and airbags helps prevent TBIs by stabilizing the head in a crash.

Sports-Related Injuries:

Contact sports like football, boxing, hockey, and rugby lead to many TBIs yearly. The accelerations and collisions during play can shake and jolt the brain. Players may also suffer blows to the head from equipment, balls, other athletes, or contact with playing surfaces. Non-contact sports like cycling, skiing, and snowboarding similarly pose TBI risks from falls and crashes. Proper protective gear and adherence to safety rules mitigate risks.

Violence/Assault:

Acts of violence are a common cause of TBI, especially among adolescents and young adults. Assaults involving blunt-force trauma, shaking of the head, or strangulation can inflict closed-head injuries. Gunshot wounds and stab injuries often produce more severe, penetrating TBIs. The consequences of violence-related TBIs extend beyond just medical issues; they pose significant psychological, social, and financial burdens on victims.

Risk Factors for Traumatic Brain Injury

While traumatic brain injuries (TBIs) can happen to anyone, certain risk factors increase their susceptibility. Understanding these risk factors enables individuals to take preventative measures and helps clinicians provide effective counseling. Major risk factors that raise the chances of suffering a TBI include:

Age:
Very young and very old individuals face a higher TBI risk. Children 0–4 years old commonly sustain TBIs from falls and abuse. Adolescents and young adults 15–24 years old incur many TBIs through falls, car accidents, sports injuries, and violence. Adults 75 years and older suffer high rates of TBI from falls due to age-related decline in vision, balance, and bone strength.

Gender:
Males face around twice the risk of TBIs compared to females. Testosterone levels, societal norms of perceived invincibility, and greater rates of participation in contact sports contribute to higher

TBI rates among men and boys. However, women still comprise nearly 40% of TBI cases annually.

Prior concussion:
Suffering any prior concussion substantially increases susceptibility to subsequent concussions and TBIs. Each concussion accumulates effects on the brain that lower its injury threshold. Proper management of initial concussions and gradually returning to normal activity can help mitigate risks.

Alcohol and drug use:
Intoxication greatly increases the chances of suffering a TBI through associated impairments to perception, judgment, reaction times, and balance. Alcohol use specifically plays a role in around half of all TBIs. Reducing hazardous alcohol consumption and stopping drug use lowers the risks.

Dangerous activities:
Contact sports such as cycling, motorcycling, skiing, snowboarding, and aerial gymnastics carry inherent TBI risks from collisions and falls. Even activities like trampolining and horseback riding pose some risk.

Using protective gear, training properly, avoiding stunts, and following safety rules help prevent injury.

Combat exposure:

Military personnel engaged in active combat face an elevated risk of sustaining TBIs from explosions, crashes, blunt force trauma, and penetrating wounds. Traumatic brain injuries comprise the "signature injury" of recent conflicts, with around 20% of 2.77 million U.S. service members estimated to have suffered a TBI.

Chapter 2

Understanding the Anatomy and Function of the Brain

The Brain's Structure and Function

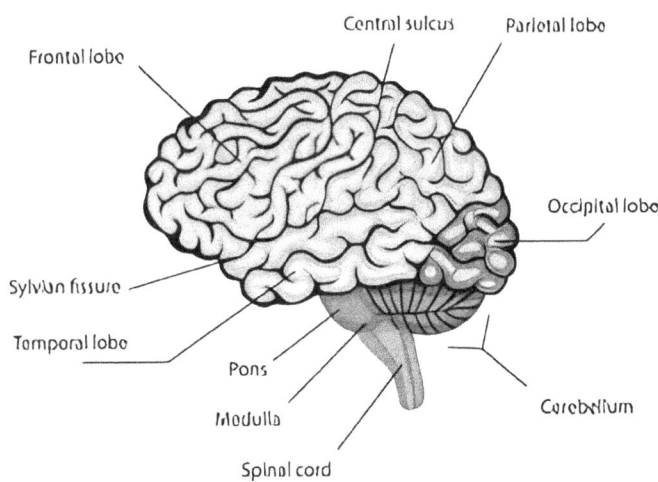

The brain is the command center of the nervous system, coordinating nearly every aspect of the human body. Understanding the brain's anatomy and function provides context for comprehending traumatic brain injury.

The brain consists of three main sections: the brainstem, cerebellum, and cerebrum. The brainstem controls crucial autonomic functions like breathing, heartbeat, and blood pressure. The cerebellum coordinates complex movements and balance. The cerebrum handles higher thinking, emotions, behavior, and sensory processing.

The cerebrum has four lobes: frontal, parietal, temporal, and occipital. The frontal lobes behind the forehead regulate executive functions, including reasoning, planning, personality, and voluntary movement. The parietal lobes process touch, temperature, pain, and body position. The temporal lobes house auditory processing, memory formation, and storage. The occipital lobes at the back contain the visual cortex.

Other important cerebrum components are the limbic system, responsible for memory and emotions, and the cortex, which handles language, consciousness, and complex thought. The cerebrum hemispheres communicate via the corpus callosum. Deeper cerebrum structures coordinate movement, orientation, arousal, motivation, learning, and habitual behaviors.

This intricate anatomy allows for the incredible computational power of the human brain. The brain is estimated to contain about 100 billion neurons interconnected by trillions of synapses. Neurons rapidly transmit electrical and chemical signals to form memories, perceptions, emotions, intentions, personalities, and all that defines a person.

Proper brain function relies on oxygen and glucose delivered by the blood to active neural tissue. The brain requires 20% of the body's oxygen despite only making up 2% of body weight. Any interruption in blood flow or oxygen supply quickly damages delicate neurons. The brain further depends on the cerebrospinal fluid that surrounds and cushions it.

The highly complex anatomy of the brain enables all cognitive, behavioral, physical, and emotional faculties. Traumatic injury disrupts structures and connections between brain regions. However, understanding the brain's geography and networks helps make sense of TBI symptoms and guides rehabilitation efforts.

How TBIs Affect Other Areas of the Brain

Traumatic brain injuries (TBIs) disrupt neural structures and connections, producing wide-ranging effects. Understanding how damage to particular brain regions relates to certain deficits helps make sense of symptoms and guide rehabilitation.

Frontal lobe injuries commonly impair judgment, self-control, planning, motivation, memory, and mood regulation. Damage may also produce personality changes like disinhibition or apathy. Movement problems can arise, too, if motor planning centers are affected.

Temporal lobe damage often harms memory consolidation and retrieval. It can make new learning difficult and blur memory formation around injury time. Speech comprehension deficits may occur with left-temporal trauma. Right-side injuries have a greater impact on visual memory and face recognition.

Parietal lobe trauma can disrupt spatial processing and internal maps of the body. This impairs balance and coordination. Injuries here also cause speech issues, an inability to focus visual attention, and an inability to process some symbolic information. Sensory deficits, touch perception problems, or altered pain sensitivity may result.

Occipital injuries produce visual field defects or blindness, depending on severity. Left occipital damage affects the right visual field and vice versa. Color, light, motion, and visual environment processing can also become impaired.

Limbic system damage affects emotion regulation, memory, and motivation. Injuries may produce dramatic mood swings, anxiety, aggression, hypersexuality, depression, or flattened emotions.

Trauma to the hippocampus specifically harms memory formation and retrieval.

Brainstem injuries vary depending on the exact location but frequently cause respiratory failure, consciousness issues, hypotension, swallowing problems, vertigo, weakness, and coordination deficits. This region controls arousal and wakefulness, too, so trauma here causes coma.

Cerebellum damage impairs fine motor skills, balance, posture, and precise movements. It disrupts muscle coordination and control of tone, leaving movements jerky and unsteady. Damage can also impact some cognitive functions, like attention and language.

Chapter 3

Symptoms and Diagnosis

Common Physical Symptoms After a TBI

Traumatic brain injuries (TBIs) often produce an array of physical symptoms and changes that can persist long after the initial injury. Understanding the most frequent physical effects helps individuals know what to expect and when to seek medical assistance. Three common physical symptoms following a TBI are headaches, dizziness, and fatigue or sleep disturbances.

Headaches:
Recurrent headaches are one of the most common and debilitating post-TBI symptoms. Over 90% of

individuals experience headaches in the first days and weeks after an injury. TBI headaches result from trauma to cranial structures, central pain network dysfunction, and increased neural excitability.

Post-TBI headaches can involve migraine features like nausea or light or noise sensitivity. They range from mild to excruciating. Headache pain may worsen with exertion, stress, or cognitive demands. Migraine, tension, or cervicogenic headache types are most common. Headaches often last over a year but usually improve with time.

Dizziness:

Dizziness affects around 80% of people after a moderate-to-severe TBI. It stems from trauma to balance centers and pathways in the brain that coordinate the vestibular system, vision, and proprioception. Dizziness may manifest as lightheadedness, vertigo, or feelings of swaying. Moving quickly often exacerbates symptoms.

Fatigue/Sleep Disturbances:

Excessive fatigue and insomnia frequently follow TBIs as well—fatigue results from increased effort for cognitive tasks, impaired sleep, and metabolic changes. Sleep cycle disruptions and the loss of restorative sleep are also common. Conditions like sleep apnea may develop post-injury, too. Managing sleep hygiene is essential for rehabilitation.

Common Cognitive Symptoms Following a TBI

Traumatic brain injuries frequently disrupt cognitive processes and lead to ongoing issues with thinking, memory, concentration, and other mental faculties. Two of the most common cognitive symptoms following TBI are memory loss and difficulty concentrating or focusing.

Memory Loss:
Memory problems are one of the hallmark deficits after TBI. Both short-term memory formation and long-term memory access become impaired. Memory loss ranges from mild forgetfulness to profound amnesia, depending on the severity and location of the injury.

Short-term memory loss causes issues with learning new information and retaining recent events. Anterograde amnesia, or the inability to form new memories, may occur. Long-term memory deficits make accessing recollections from before the injury difficult. Retrograde amnesia can erase memories from years prior.

Memory loss results from damage to temporal lobe structures like the hippocampus or diffuse axonal injuries that disrupt connections between brain regions. Memory typically improves over the first year but may have lasting effects.

Difficulty Concentrating/Focusing:

Sustaining attention and concentration on tasks is frequently challenging after a TBI. Processing speed slows, while mental fatigue sets in quickly on cognitive tasks. Switching between tasks or being distracted is difficult.

Attention deficits stem from diffuse damage to the brain networks that coordinate focus and processing. Slowed speed relates to axonal injuries. Fatigue arises from the extra effort required to complete tasks.

Attention and concentration impairments make conversations, reading, work/school duties, and other everyday activities more difficult. Strategies like minimizing distractions, allowing more time, and dividing tasks into smaller steps can help overcome these issues.

Common Behavioral and Emotional Symptoms Following a TBI

In addition to physical and cognitive changes, traumatic brain injuries (TBIs) often result in behavioral and emotional symptoms that affect mood, personality, and social functioning. Two examples of frequent behavioral and emotional issues after TBI are mood swings or irritability and depression or anxiety.

Mood Swings/Irritability:

Rapid mood swings and irritability are common after a TBI causes damage to brain regions that regulate emotions and behavior. Injury to the frontal lobes reduces self-control, while limbic system damage causes excessive emotional reactions.

Mood swings may involve dramatic shifts from laughing to crying to anger in quick succession. Irritability often presents as a low frustration tolerance, frequent temper outbursts, and increased agitation in response to stressors.

These issues strain relationships with family, friends, and caregivers. Developing coping strategies and having open communication helps manage Symptoms, which usually improve over time but may have lasting impacts on personality.

Depression/Anxiety:

Depression affects over half of TBI survivors in the first year, while anxiety issues impact nearly three-quarters. Depression relates to adjustment difficulties, pain, cognitive problems, and neurochemical changes. Anxiety often centers on functional losses and uncertainty for the future.

Symptoms of depression include persistent low mood, loss of enjoyment, changes in sleep or appetite, low energy, and thoughts of worthlessness. Anxiety manifests through obsessive worry, panic attacks, and avoidance behaviors.

Assessment by a neuropsychologist helps identify mood disorders that need treatment. Counseling, medication, lifestyle changes, and support groups can all help manage depression and anxiety. Persistent mental health issues may necessitate long-term care.

Diagnostic Procedures for a TBI

When a traumatic brain injury (TBI) is suspected, prompt diagnostic testing helps determine the presence and severity of the injury. This facilitates appropriate acute treatment and enables the prediction of likely outcomes. Common diagnostic procedures for evaluating TBI include:

1. **Neurological exam:** Tests like pupil reaction, movement and sensation, balance, speech, and cognitive function help detect neurological deficits indicating TBI.

2. **Head CT scan:** This provides visualization of skull fractures, bleeding or swelling in the brain, and contusions. It is the standard initial test for determining structural damage from TBI.

3. **Head MRI:** Magnetic resonance imaging offers more detailed views of brain structures and networks than CT scans. This helps assess axonal shearing injuries and small contusions that can influence function.

4. **Functional MRI:** Used primarily in research, fMRI detects changes in blood oxygenation related to neural activity in different brain regions. This sheds light on network disruptions.

5. **EEG:** Electroencephalography records electrical activity in the brain. It can identify seizures and aid the prognosis for coma patients by looking for signs of intact networks.

6. **Neuropsychological testing:** Formal pencil and paper tests evaluate areas like memory, executive function, attention, information processing speed, language skills, spatial abilities, and mood. Results help determine specific deficits.

7. **Serum biomarkers:** Levels of proteins like GFAP, UCH-L1, SBDPs, and S100B in the blood can indicate TBI severity and the

prognosis for recovery based on the extent of cellular damage.

Combining multiple modalities provides the clearest diagnostic picture of structural damage, functional impairments, and projected outcomes following TBI. For mild cases, a neurological exam and cognitive testing may suffice. Severe TBI warrants utilizing multiple neuroimaging techniques, EEG, and biomarker tests. Ongoing assessments during rehabilitation are key to gauging recovery progress.

Chapter 4

Treatment Options for Individuals with Traumatic Brain Injury (TBI)

Multidisciplinary Treatment Approach

Due to the complex and variable effects of traumatic brain injury (TBI), a coordinated, multidisciplinary approach is essential for rehabilitation and maximizing outcomes. This involves a team of professionals with expertise spanning the many facets of function affected by TBI. Key members of a multidisciplinary TBI treatment team include:

1. **Physicians (neurologists):** Provide medical management, such as monitoring for secondary

complications, prescribing medications, and performing follow-up procedures as needed.

2. **Rehabilitation nurses:** Handle day-to-day care needs, educate on health management, and monitor progress.

3. **Physical therapists:** Improve mobility, gait, balance, and coordination through therapeutic exercises and activities.

4. **Occupational therapists:** Increase independence with daily tasks like self-care, household duties, job skills, and driving readiness through functional retraining.

5. **Speech-language pathologists:** Work on communication disorders, cognitive-linguistic deficits, and swallowing difficulties through oral motor and speech rehabilitation.

6. **Neuropsychologists:** Assess and treat cognitive, behavioral, and emotional issues using counseling, cognitive rehabilitation strategies, and therapies like CBT.

7. **Recreation therapists:** Teach adaptive sports and leisure activities that improve quality of life and community participation.

8. **Case managers:** Coordinate care plans, services, equipment needs, discharge preparations, and transition to outpatient rehabilitation.

With regular team meetings and communication, each provider offers expertise to optimize rehabilitation. This addresses the full spectrum of medical, physical, cognitive, emotional, and daily living needs. It also allows for adjusting strategies based on progress and setbacks.

Active involvement of patients and families is critical, too. Setting collaborative goals and communicating challenges and successes helps the team tailor efforts. Peer support programs are also a key component of holistic TBI rehabilitation.

The multidisciplinary approach recognizes that recovery from TBI depends on more than just medical treatment. Combining comprehensive services, this model delivers integrated care for the best functional results.

Rehabilitation Options

Rehabilitation is crucial for relearning skills, regaining independence, and improving quality of life after a traumatic brain injury (TBI). While an integrated multidisciplinary approach is ideal, common therapeutic services can aid recovery when utilized individually. Key rehabilitation options for TBI include physical, occupational, and speech therapy.

Physical Therapy:

Physical therapy aims to restore mobility, strength, balance, and coordination impaired by TBI. Exercises focus on gross motor skills like sitting, standing, walking, and climbing stairs. Therapists design custom exercise programs to improve muscle control, posture, stamina, and function.

Techniques like tilt tables, suspension therapy, and aquatic exercises help develop strength and retrain movement. Balance and vertigo issues are addressed through gaze stabilization and proprioceptive retraining exercises. Mobility aids, orthotics, and other equipment may assist in recovery.

Occupational Therapy:

Occupational therapy helps rebuild skills needed for everyday activities and tasks like self-care, household duties, driving, school activities, and work. Therapists identify barriers to independence and employ exercises, adaptive techniques, and devices to overcome them.

Cognitive rehabilitation strategies teach ways to manage memory, attention, planning, and organization issues. Computer-based programs aim to improve visual processing speed and reasoning deficits, too. The goal is to build skills for maximum independence.

Speech Therapy:

Speech therapy targets communication disorders, cognitive-linguistic problems, and swallowing difficulties stemming from TBI. Exercises strengthen oral motor control and breathing for clearer speech. Therapists help rebuild language processing and production skills like conversation, reading, and writing.

For swallowing problems, therapists teach compensatory strategies and exercises to improve the safety and efficiency of swallowing. Alternative communication devices may be recommended if verbal abilities remain limited.

Medications to Manage Symptoms

Medications often play a supportive role in managing common symptoms and issues following a traumatic brain injury (TBI). While medicines do not directly cure deficits, they help control symptoms that interfere with daily functioning and quality of life. Typical medications for TBI symptoms include pain relievers, antidepressants, anxiolytics, and stimulants.

Pain Management:
Medications help relieve frequent headaches, musculoskeletal pain, and other sources of chronic pain post-TBI. Over-the-counter pain relievers like acetaminophen, ibuprofen, and naproxen are commonly used for mild pain. Prescription opioids or nerve pain medications may be needed for more severe pain.

Antidepressants/Anxiolytics:

Antidepressants often aid in managing depression and anxiety, as well as sleep issues after TBI. Selective serotonin reuptake inhibitors like sertraline, fluoxetine, and citalopram tend to be the first choices, given their relative safety and efficacy. Other types, like tricyclics or SNRIs, may also help.

Anti-anxiety drugs such as benzodiazepines offer short-term relief from anxiety but require close monitoring due to their risks. Long-term medications like buspirone may be safer options for ongoing anxiety issues post-TBI.

Stimulants:

Stimulant medications like methylphenidate, dextroamphetamine, and modafinil counteract mental fatigue and cognitive dysfunction in some TBI cases. They act by increasing levels of dopamine and norepinephrine to enhance alertness, concentration, and focus. Stimulants may support rehabilitation efforts and day-to-day functioning.

However, no medications are universally effective for all individuals with TBI. A tailored approach weighing potential benefits and side effect risks is needed, along with close monitoring and dosage adjustments. Non-pharmacological strategies should be utilized as well to promote healing and independence.

Supportive Therapies for Individuals Recovering from a TBI

In addition to formal rehabilitation, various supportive therapies and tools significantly aid the healing and adaptation process following a traumatic brain injury (TBI). Supportive options like counseling, nutritional support, and assistive devices and equipment empower individuals to participate actively in their recovery.

Counseling:

Psychotherapy helps many cope with emotional changes and mental health issues post-TBI, like depression, anxiety, anger, and grief. Cognitive behavioral therapy, in particular, teaches strategies to regulate emotions, manage stress, improve thought patterns, and develop healthy behaviors. Joining support groups provides connections.

Nutritional Support:

Optimal nutrition supports the energy demands of brain healing and aids cognitive function. Complex carbohydrates, lean proteins, omega-3s, colorful fruits and vegetables, and staying hydrated maintain brain health. Avoiding refined sugars, saturated fats, and stimulants is recommended. Nutritional counseling ensures adequate intake.

Assistive Devices/Equipment:

Devices that adapt to the environment enable greater safety and independence with daily tasks. Grab bars, shower seats, dressing aids, and adapted cooking utensils facilitate self-care. Electronic aids like reminders, communication devices, audio recordings, and GPS trackers support memory and orientation.

Mobility devices, including canes, walkers, wheelchairs, or orthotics, allow safer movement and reduce fall risks. Adaptive driving equipment helps manage visual, motor, and cognitive issues behind the wheel. Assistive technologies should align with current and future needs.

Chapter 5

Management Strategies for Families and Caregivers

The Impact of TBI on Loved Ones

When an individual close to you suffers a traumatic brain injury, the effects extend far beyond just the survivor. TBI profoundly impacts family members and caregivers emotionally, physically, socially, and financially. Understanding these potential impacts empowers loved ones to manage challenges and maintain their health.

A TBI often thrusts families suddenly into a caregiving role, which can take a major physical and emotional toll over time. Witnessing personality changes, cognitive deficits, and loss of independence in a loved one is also devastating. Caregivers frequently report persistent anxiety, depression, grief, and fatigue.

TBI survivors may exhibit behavioral symptoms like aggression, impulsivity, or emotional volatility stemming from the injury. Coping with these ongoing issues strains relationships between the survivor and family members. Partners may feel like they have lost the person they once knew.

Life becomes dominated by medical care, rehabilitation, and uncertainty for the future. Families spend less time with friends or on personal interests. Caregivers have higher risks of illness. Jobs, finances, and family roles are disrupted. These effects can last months or years, depending on the severity of the injury.

However, supports like respite care, counseling, and joining support communities help sustain caregiver health and the family unit. Celebrating small wins in recovery brings hope. Families can adjust to a new normal with time, adaptation, and grief counseling.

Explaining TBI effects to children, leveraging extended family for support, and taking breaks to prevent burnout. Open communication and a team approach to care with professionals, the survivor, and the family are beneficial, too. Maintaining personal health and sources of joy enables being the best possible caregiver.

The impacts of TBI extend far beyond the survivor alone. However, awareness of common challenges means families can take steps to care for themselves and adapt together. With compassion, patience, education, support, and hope, loved ones can manage the journey to a new normal.

Coping Mechanisms for Caregivers of Individuals with Traumatic Brain Injury

Caring for someone with a traumatic brain injury (TBI) brings profound challenges. Utilizing positive coping strategies helps caregivers manage stress and avoid burnout. Two important coping mechanisms for TBI caregivers are seeking support from others and practicing self-care.

Seeking Support:

Support from others provides caregivers with connection, encouragement, and practical advice. Support groups allow learning from those with shared experiences. Counseling aids in processing emotions. Respite care offers breaks.

Online communities, through sites like BrainLine.org, facilitate finding support. Local brain injury associations have in-person programs and mentors. Support from family, friends, religious communities, or peer mentors is helpful too.

Connecting with the rehabilitation team provides education and links to resources. Being involved in the survivor's therapies also offers encouragement. Support groups empower caregivers to be most effective in their roles.

Practicing Self-Care:

Making personal health and well-being a priority is also key. Self-care prevents exhaustion and sustains the ability to support the survivor. Key aspects include:

- Taking breaks and sharing duties with other family and friends,
- Maintaining social connections and enjoyable hobbies,
- Engaging in stress relief activities like therapy, meditation, yoga, and journaling,
- Exercising and eating healthy to manage energy,
- Getting adequate sleep to stay refreshed
- Setting boundaries and not taking on too much
- Celebrating progress and positive moments of connection

Seeking help when needed and saying "no" prevents burnout. Respite care, adult day programs, or in-home assistants periodically provide rest. Self-care maintains resilience to better serve the survivor in the long term.

Tips for Families and Caregivers on Creating a Supportive Environment for Individuals with TBI

A supportive home environment optimizes function and quality of life for individuals with TBI. Family members and caregivers play a key role in setting up the living space, establishing routines, facilitating engagement, and interacting compassionately. Useful tips include:

- Maintaining structure through planning, calendars, and schedules. Help manage time and sequence tasks. Set reminders for everything from chores to medications. Consistency and step-by-step guides aid independence.

- Adapt the home for accessibility, safety, and convenience by installing grab bars, stair railings, adequate lighting, easy-open handles, ramps, or first-floor living space. Reduce clutter and tripping hazards.

- Use notes, signs, labels, and written instructions to guide activities if memory, communication, or comprehension are impaired. Auditory reminders and smart devices can cue as well. Provide notebooks to organize information.

- Adjust tasks and routines to match the person's capabilities, energy level, and interests—scale activities from simple to complex. Recognize small wins and celebrate incremental progress.

- Stimulate cognitive skills through puzzles, games, crafts, or apps. Engage in hobbies, social interactions, and leisure pursuits they enjoy. Avoid sensory overload.

- Be patient, flexible, and understanding when providing care and support. Respond with empathy, not criticism, to personality changes. Foster independence, but help when needed.

- Educate family and friends on interacting constructively. Maintain social connections that enrich the quality of life. Offer sincere encouragement and praise. Find appropriate peer support.

- Collaborate on setting goals, making decisions, and monitoring progress. Offer choices and respect preferences to support autonomy. Provide honest feedback sensitively.

With some adaptations and compassionate communication, the home can become a sanctuary that enables continued development. Support people with TBI in pursuing their interests and meaningfully contributing to family life.

Chapter 6

Long-Term Effects and Prognosis

Potential Long-Term Effects of TBI

While some symptoms resolve quickly, TBI can also result in persisting physical, cognitive, emotional, and functional impairments over months or years. Understanding common long-term effects helps survivors, families, and professionals plan rehabilitation and life adjustments.

Physical Effects:
Frequent physical effects include chronic headaches, vertigo, sleep disorders, sensory changes like photophobia or tinnitus, chronic pain, weakness or spasticity, seizures, and an increased risk for

neurodegenerative diseases. Some may have permanent vision or hearing loss, speech disabilities, or mobility impairments, depending on the injury location.

Cognitive and Emotional Effects:

Cognitive deficits commonly involve attention, concentration, memory, information processing speed, judgment, and executive functioning. These interfere with learning and decision-making. Emotional effects like depression, anxiety, aggression, impulsivity, and personality changes are common as well. Social cognition and behavior may be impacted.

Impact on Daily Life:

Ongoing cognitive and physical limitations impede independence in self-care, household duties, employment, schoolwork, driving, sports, and recreational activities. Assistance may be needed for decision-making in finances, healthcare, and legal matters. Relationships, family roles, and social life can suffer without support.

However, the trajectory over the first year post-injury helps predict long-term outcomes. Participating in rehabilitation and implementing recommended therapies and lifestyle changes help some regain prior capabilities. Supportive technologies and accommodations further aid independence. With realistic expectations and support, many adapt and enjoy quality of life.

The Prognosis for Recovery After TBI and Life Afterwards

The Recovery prognosis varies widely between individuals based on injury characteristics and response to rehabilitation. While predicting exact outcomes is difficult, certain factors affect the overall recovery potential. With proper support, many can still enjoy fulfilling lives post-TBI.

Factors Affecting Recovery:

Injury severity correlates with recovery extent and timeline. Mild TBIs often resolve in weeks or months with supportive care. Moderate to severe TBIs have prolonged recovery periods and a higher disability risk. Repeated injuries have compound effects.

Age impacts plasticity, too. Children have greater potential for neural rewiring than older adults. However, early injuries may still alter development. Pre-injury health and cognitive reserves also play a role. Co-occurring conditions like stroke or neurological disorders can hamper healing.

Response to early treatment and engagement with rehabilitation programs provide major prognostic information. Following recommendations maximizes the potential for gains. Ongoing direct therapy and at-home exercise for months or years are often beneficial.

Life After Traumatic Brain Injury:

With rehabilitation, assistive technologies, accommodations, and lifestyle adjustments, many survivors return to independent living and working. Supportive communities, friendships, family relationships, and purposeful activities enrich life.

For moderate-to-severe injuries, greater dependence on others for care may persist. However, focusing on strengths and social connections improves coping. Survivors find meaning through advocacy, educating others, creative pursuits, or volunteering. Hope, personal growth, and life purpose can emerge from the recovery journey.

While disabilities may remain, outlook and effort positively influence the quality of life after TBI. Healing over time, celebrating progress, receiving support, and finding purpose help survivors and families adapt and thrive despite changes wrought by trauma.

Chapter 7

Prevention of Traumatic Brain Injury

Education and Awareness about TBI

A greater public understanding of TBI is the foundation for prevention efforts. Education raises awareness of risks, empowers protective actions, and fosters a culture of TBI prevention. Key knowledge areas to promote include:

1. **Signs, symptoms, and potential consequences of TBI:** Broad education on recognizing brain injury and seeking prompt care improves outcomes. Understanding common post-TBI issues like cognitive deficits,

personality changes, and chronic health problems encourages support.

2. **Situations that typically cause TBI:** Highlighting leading causes like falls, motor vehicle crashes, sports and recreation, and violence informs the public where prevention should be targeted. Education on specific risks empowers avoidance.

3. **Populations most vulnerable to TBI:** Awareness of increased risks among children, teens, older adults, certain athletes, and military personnel promotes focused prevention initiatives in these groups. This includes tailored education.

4. **The cumulative effects of repeated mild TBIs:** Explaining how repetitive sub-concussive and concussive injuries compound over time, increasing susceptibility to severe TBI and neurodegeneration inspires protective action.

5. **Best practices for TBI prevention and response:** Sharing proven prevention tips like wearing seatbelts and helmets, fall-proofing

homes, and detecting concussion signs ensures people have actionable strategies for safety.

Knowledge transforms behaviors and social norms. Pairing education with policy changes and safety technology advances can dramatically reduce TBI incidence through the widespread adoption of preventative practices. All have roles in spreading awareness: health professionals, schools, government agencies, community organizations, and the media. Education establishes a shared responsibility for TBI prevention.

Precautions to Prevent Accidents and Injuries

While not always preventable, proactive measures greatly reduce the chances of sustaining a traumatic brain injury (TBI). Safety steps like wearing helmets, using seatbelts, and preventing concussions in sports minimize key injury risks.

Helmet Safety:

Helmets protect against TBI from falls, collisions, and other head impacts during activities like bicycling, motorcycling, horseback riding, skiing/snowboarding, construction work, and military duty. Models meeting safety standards reduce the force transferred to the head by up to 88%.

Proper helmet fit and consistent use are crucial. Beyond motor vehicle use, helmets should be worn for recreation as well. Multi-directional impacts warrant helmets over just headbands. As helmet materials degrade with age, replace them regularly.

Seatbelt Use:

Wearing seatbelts saves lives and prevents TBI in a motor vehicle accident. Belts distribute crash forces across strong torso bones rather than directly to the head and brain. Seatbelts also reduce ejection risk and protect passengers from striking the interior during collisions.

Seatbelt use is required by law. Advanced designs like shoulder straps and pre-tensioners provide further protection. Children must use age- or size-appropriate restraints. Proper seatbelt habits prevent major TBI risks from driving.

Concussion Prevention in Sports:

Given the higher rates of repetitive TBIs from contact sports, prevention is critical. Fair play, respecting rules, avoiding dangerous techniques like spear tackling or checks to the head, and banning helmet-first contact help protect athletes.

For suspected concussions, immediate removal from play and evaluation using validated assessment tools like SCAT-5 aid recovery before further activity. Gradual return to sport follows recovery stages only with medical clearance. Protective equipment should meet current safety standards, too. Players, coaches, officials, and leagues all promote safety.

Chapter 8

Resources for Individuals with TBI and their Families

TBI Support Groups for Survivors and Families

Support groups connect individuals and families affected by TBI to share experiences, find emotional support, and exchange practical advice for navigating recovery. They provide a sense of community and empowerment. Useful support groups include:

1. **Brain Injury Association Support Groups:** With a network of state chapters and local groups, the Brain Injury Association hosts in-person and virtual support groups facilitated

by professionals. Groups are tailored for survivors, caregivers, or family members.

2. **TBI CAMP:** TBI Consumer Camps bring together survivors annually for recreational therapy, peer mentoring, and workshops on living skills. Social connections motivate continued progress.

3. **TBI Peer-to-Peer Support:** One-on-one mentoring from trained support partners with personal TBI experience provides ongoing emotional support and encouragement.

4. **TBI Caregivers Support Group:** Connecting with fellow caregivers helps them process challenges, gain insights, and find encouragement. Sharing needs and taking breaks improves well-being.

5. **Online TBI Support Communities:** Websites like BrainLine.org and apps like MyTBIenable allow users to exchange advice anytime. Discussion boards foster connections among people with diverse backgrounds and injury severity.

6. **Local Hospital & Rehab Center Groups:** Many leading rehabilitation providers host support groups for former patients and their families. These build a community of nearby people who understand the experience.

7. **Faith community, recreational, and activity groups:** Supportive social connections, tailored activities, and a sense of belonging also aid well-being after TBI.

TBI support groups reduce isolation and provide authentic understanding from shared experiences. They empower survivors and families through relationships, role models, and exchanging knowledge on recovery.

Outpatient Services Following a TBI

Outpatient rehabilitation programs help continue the recovery gains made in the hospital after sustaining a TBI. Ongoing therapies, medical management, and support services aid the transition to home and community life. Useful outpatient services include:

1. **Physical, occupational, and speech therapy:** Address persistent mobility, self-care, communication, and swallowing deficits through exercises and functional retraining. It helps rebuild skills for independence.

2. **Cognitive rehabilitation:** Uses strategies like computer training programs and group classes to improve attention, memory, planning, reasoning, and processing speed to support daily activities.

3. **Neuropsychological services:** Assess residual cognitive, behavioral, and emotional deficits. Provides counseling, biofeedback, and cognitive-behavioral therapy for issues like depression, anxiety, and anger management.

4. **Case management:** Assists with care coordination, equipment acquisition, home accessibility modifications, vehicle adaptations, pursuing benefits and legal claims, and transitioning back to school or work.

5. **Recreational therapy:** Adapts leisure activities, provides community reintegration

skills training, and teaches compensatory strategies to improve quality of life—fostering social connections.

6. **Drug & alcohol rehabilitation:** Addresses substance abuse issues stemming from TBI through counseling, peer support, and medication-assisted treatment when necessary. Prevents complications.

7. **Chronic pain programs:** Combine physical therapy, medications, injections, counseling, relaxation techniques, and lifestyle changes to help manage ongoing headaches, muscle pain, or other sources of chronic pain after TBI.

8. **Neurology follow-up:** Monitors seizure risk, regulates medications for optimal benefit, and manages associated neurological conditions impacting recoveries like stroke or migraine. Provides continuity after hospital care.

Local Organizations and Resources that Support Individuals with TBI and Their Families

In addition to treatment providers, various local community organizations, agencies, and services assist people impacted by TBI. Connecting with local resources provides long-term support, education, advocacy, and the tools to maximize quality of life. Useful local options to explore include:

1. **Brain Injury Associations:** State chapters and local support groups provide education, peer mentoring, rehabilitation guidance, and advocacy. Chapters assist with locating counseling, legal aid, housing, and employment programs.

2. **Independent Living Centers:** Offer skills training, counseling, advocacy, assistive technology grants, and home modification funding to enhance independence for people with disabilities.

3. **Area Agencies on Aging:** Coordinate in-home support services, transportation, meal

programs, day centers, and caregiver counseling. Benefits consulting assists older adult TBI survivors.

4. **Centers for Independent Living:** Nonprofits providing advocacy, skills training, counseling, and resources to aid community integration and self-sufficiency after disability. Peers help the newly injured.

5. **Local United Way:** Provides information, directs people to specialized support programs, and may offer emergency funds for TBI-related needs like assistive equipment, therapy co-pays, or vehicle modifications.

6. **Public Libraries:** Offer free computers/internet, assistive technology, audiobooks, accessibility apps, health programs, study spaces, and extended time on tasks. Help re-establish community connections.

7. **Local Support Groups:** Connect with other TBI survivors and caregivers for mutual understanding, advice, encouragement, and friendship. Support one another in adjusting.

Check national directories and local health providers for specialized brain injury services nearby. County and municipal governments may have dedicated disability and senior services offices, too—maximal local support.

Online Resources that Support Individuals with TBI and Their Families

The internet provides many resources to supplement medical care and community support for those affected by TBI. Online resources offer convenience, connections, encouragement, and specialized information at one's fingertips. Helpful online options include:

1. **BrainLine.org:** A leading web resource from TBI experts covering injury basics, coping strategies, community supports, assistive technology, advocacy, and current research. Offers webinars and moderates online support communities.

2. **MyTBI.org:** Provides personalized, interactive guides to TBI recovery through

video courses, assessment tools, health tracking, and expert access. Developed with leading rehabilitation centers.

3. **TBITrust.org:** Features a comprehensive, evidence-based video series on the TBI recovery journey and community stories. Provides e-books, life skills courses, and expert services.

4. **Specialized sites like TBINet.org, Neuroskills.com, and TBICentral.com:** Offer webinars, blogs, support groups, rehabilitation tips, and provider/service locators. Help navigate complex TBI issues.

5. **TBI Facebook Groups:** Connect with others affected by TBI for real-time advice, emotional support, inspiration, and friendship. Groups exist for survivors, caregivers, teens, athletes, veterans, and spouses.

6. **YouTube channels from therapists and survivors:** Provide free video tutorials on therapy exercises, assistive techniques for daily tasks, device reviews, advocacy advice, and personal recovery journeys.

7. **Government and nonprofit sites like CDC.gov/TBI, MayoClinic.org, and NIH.gov/TBI:** Offer comprehensive medical information and the latest research findings to educate on injury impacts and treatments.

The internet expands knowledge, community, and hope after TBI. Online tools aid recovery and life enrichment for survivors and their families from any location.

Conclusion

Traumatic brain injury (TBI) is a complex health condition that causes sudden, profound life disruption. However, with education, support, and proper rehabilitation, many individuals experience recovery and adaptation after TBI. Key takeaways include:

- TBI arises from external forces on the brain through events like falls, crashes, sports, and violence. Effects range from mild concussions to severe disabilities based on injury characteristics.
- Understanding TBI empowers those affected to seek appropriate care, set expectations, advocate for their needs, and lower future risks. Knowledge guides families in providing compassionate support as well.

- TBI often produces lasting cognitive, physical, emotional, and daily living challenges stemming from diffuse brain network and structure damage. Ongoing symptom management and lifestyle adjustments are frequently needed.

- Rehabilitation through physical, occupational, speech, recreation, and counseling therapies aims to redevelop skills and independence. Medications, devices, nutrition, and home modifications further support function.

- Creating a structured, positive environment and maintaining family relationships, social connections, meaningful activities, and a sense of purpose help adapt and enhance the quality of life after TBI.

- Education, safety practices, responsible sports participation, and addressing issues like substance abuse play key roles in preventing TBIs at individual and societal levels. Protective steps save lives and reduce injury risks.

- TBI resilience depends on comprehensive care, realistic hope, self-advocacy, social support, development of new meaning, and tailored life enrichment. Survivors and their families can craft fulfilling lives after injury with patience and guidance.

The Importance of Seeking Timely Medical Attention After a Head Injury

Any head injury causing concerning symptoms, even mild ones, warrants urgent medical evaluation to determine if a TBI occurred and avoid potentially serious consequences. Timely diagnosis and early interventions improve outcomes after TBI.

Seeking immediate emergency care is crucial with signs like loss of consciousness, seizure, repeated vomiting, worsening headache, inability to awaken, or profound confusion. Rapid treatment may prevent secondary brain damage from uncontrolled bleeding, swelling, or changes in oxygen or blood flow.

Ongoing monitoring in the hospital for complications like swelling, fluid buildup, cerebral vasospasm, seizures, and hydrocephalus can be lifesaving. Delaying care risks irreversible damage or even death with severe TBIs.

However, even seemingly mild head blows require evaluation, as life-long disabilities may result from undiagnosed concussions. Repeated, untreated concussions compound harm to the brain. A medical professional can assess subtle signs and utilize imaging and cognitive testing to identify TBI.

Early rehabilitation interventions promote neuronal healing and recovery. Occupational, physical, speech, and cognitive therapies restore function after a diagnosed injury. Delay prolongs struggles with cognition, coordination, and daily living skills.

Additionally, a medical record of injury, symptoms, and treatments supports any future claims with health insurance, disability benefits, legal proceedings, school accommodations, or workplace modifications as lingering effects emerge.

Overall, seeking prompt medical care maximizes the chances of the best possible recovery and long-term outcomes after any TBI severity. Do not brush off a head blow, assuming one needs to "shake it off." Protect your brain health and quality of life by getting evaluated when injuries occur and following all recommended treatments.

The Importance of Continuous Learning About Traumatic Brain Injury (TBI)

Understanding TBI is lifelong as new research continually emerges. For individuals affected, families, and medical providers, keeping up-to-date through reputable sources ensures access to evidence-based information on injury causes, treatments, management strategies, and resources.

Reliable resources for ongoing TBI education include the following:

- Brain injury associations like BrainLine.org, MyBrainInjury.com, and the American Association of Neurological Surgeons.
- Academic institutions such as medical schools and rehabilitation research centers.

- Government agencies like the CDC's Injury Center and the NIH's National Institute on Disability, Independent Living, and Rehabilitation Research.
- Supportive nonprofits like the Brain Injury Research Institute and the International Brain Injury Association.
- Leading medical journals such as The Journal of Head Trauma Rehabilitation, Neurology, Journal of Neurotrauma, and Brain Injury.
- Respected hospitals and rehabilitation facilities like Craig Hospital, Shirley Ryan AbilityLab, Mayo Clinic, and Boston University CTE Center.

Staying up-to-date empowers individuals with TBI and their families to be active and informed participants in care decisions. Current knowledge aids discussions with medical teams. For professionals, continuing education ensures the delivery of best practices that maximize patient outcomes and improve quality of life.

Sustained learning also enables those affected by TBI to access the latest support. New rehabilitation techniques, therapies, medications, devices, disability laws, and home modification technologies continuously emerge. Updated awareness connects people to new options for recovery assistance.

Make continuing education on TBI through reputable sources a lifelong habit. Be an advocate for your care and help others by sharing current knowledge. With learning and growth, a hopeful future unfolds.

Final Thoughts on the Positive Impact of Understanding (TBI)

When suddenly faced with TBI, arming oneself with knowledge provides a foundation of clarity and empowerment. Comprehending the basics of injury causes, symptoms, treatments, and demonstrated paths forward lights the way. While the road to recovery has its challenges, understanding brings hope.

For individuals with TBI, learning about your condition allows for setting reasonable expectations and advocating for your needs during care. You can make informed decisions on therapies, services, and lifestyle changes to support your recovery. Knowing recovery is a journey; you can focus on celebrating small daily wins.

Understanding your deficits also enables you to adopt strategies and technologies to enhance your independence in daily life. Knowledge empowers asking for accommodations at school or work as well. Being your best advocate is key to getting quality care and living life fully after TBI.

For family members, understanding grounds you to be a compassionate support system. Learning about typical TBI effects and needs equips you to create an optimal healing environment. Knowing what your loved one is experiencing allows you to encourage them through challenges.

Friends also play a critical role when they comprehend the impacts of TBI. Your empathetic support aids recovery and enriches daily life through meaningful shared activities. With understanding, you can provide needed encouragement while seeing your friend as their same wonderful self, not just defined by injury.

For all affected by or close to someone with TBI, make learning a priority. Let information guide you on this journey of hope. Have patience, celebrate progress, find purpose in each day, and believe in greater healing ahead. The human brain and spirit have incredible resilience. Understanding TBI builds the foundation to continue living a fulfilling life.